5 STEPS BABY SLEEP SOLUTION

SAVE TIME, TEARS & HELP YOUR BABY TO SLEEP DEEPLY THROUGH THE NIGHT

PATRICK BRADLEY

Legal & Disclaimer

The information contained in this book and its contents is not designed to replace or take the place of any form of medical or professional advice; and is not meant to replace the need for independent medical, financial, legal or other professional advice or services, as may be required. The content and information in this book have been provided for educational and entertainment purposes only.

The content and information contained in this book have been compiled from sources deemed reliable, and it is accurate to the best of the Author's knowledge, information, and belief. However, the Author cannot guarantee its accuracy and validity and cannot be held liable for any errors and/or omissions. Further, changes are periodically made to this book as and when needed. Where appropriate and/or necessary, you must consult a professional (including but not limited to your doctor, attorney, financial advisor or such other professional advisor) before using any of the suggested remedies, techniques, or information in this book.

Upon using the contents and information contained in this book, you agree to hold harmless the Author from and against any damages, costs, and expenses, including any legal fees potentially resulting from the application of any of the information provided by this book. This disclaimer applies to any loss, damages or injury caused by the use and application, whether directly or indirectly, of any advice or information presented, whether for breach of contract, tort, negligence, personal injury, criminal intent, or under any other cause of action.

You agree to accept all risks of using the information presented inside this book.

You agree that by continuing to read this book, where appropriate and/or necessary, you shall consult a professional (including but not

TABLE OF CONTENTS

INTRODUCTION

Sleep in babies is very critical especially during the first stage of their lives. It is your responsibility to make sure that your toddler gets enough sleep. Sleep aids in the growth and development of your baby.

Are you a parent who is frustrated by the sleeping pattern of your kids? Do you want to accelerate sleeping training for your kids? Are you tired of implementing bad sleeping training to your kids? Then this guide for you.

In this book, I am going to share with the secrets to use to achieve success in sleep training. For those who do not know what sleep training is; it simply the process of teaching or helping your kid to learn how to fall asleep and sleep longer.

You have heard people saying; "You will not sleep again" during baby showers. For the first few months, a baby has yet to establish a good sleeping pattern. Their sleep is confusing and inconsistent. Your baby may wake up in the middle of the night and sleep during the day. This is entirely normal, and there is no reason to be alarmed.

The good news is that it is possible to establish a predictable sleep-cycle for your kid. I will teach you how to achieve success in sleep training within five days. This will allow you and your family to enjoy a good night's sleep undisturbed.

CHAPTER 1

BABY SLEEP TRAINING IS A HOT TOPIC FOR MOST PARENTS

There is nothing as stressful as having sleepless nights because your infant doesn't sleep. This is something that makes most parents be stressful and look out for solutions. Most parents are desperate to find the best sleep training plan to help their kids get enough sleep and sleep better.

There are lots of questions that parents ask themselves. We will be trying to answer some of these questions, and we believe they this will provide a solution to the sleep training problem that most parents face.

Some parents hate to see their baby cry. Because of this, you will find out that most sleep techniques are for both parents and kids. That for example, the CIO (Cry It Out) this sleep training program is for the kid and not the parent.

Scientist argues that when the child cries, it helps in relieving stress and eventually they will fall asleep. On the other hand, as a parent, you will have to bear with the cry of your kid until they fall asleep.

Other forms of sleep training help parent and everyone else in the home to sleep. When your child is sound asleep, you will have peace of mind, and you too will fall asleep as well.

In the next section, we will be trying to answer 8 most burning questions parents ask about sleep training.

Top 8 Burning Questions Parents Ask about Their Baby's Sleep

Sleep training is not easy for most parents. This is the reason why we get so many questions about baby sleep as parents try to get varied opinion and answers to this issue. Some of the top questions baby sleep includes.

Q1. Help My Baby Won't Sleep, What Could Be the Reason?

Nothing is distressing as waking up in the middle of the night to get your baby to sleep. There are so many reasons why your baby won't sleep. This reason can either be health reasons or other factors. Mostly health reasons are the least, and other are the ones which contributed to lack of sleep.

The following are some of the reasons why your baby won't sleep: keep in mind that these are the common one there can be more.

1. Your Baby is Overtired

There is a myth that many parents believe in that when a baby is overtired, that's when they will fall asleep quickly. This is not the case; when they are super tired, they will not sleep right, and they will keep on waking up.

Make sure that your baby does not get overtired by creating a schedule where you will incorporate nap times when they show a sign of tiredness.

2. They Are Too Excited to Sleep

Also known as overstimulation; it means that your kid is in an environment which is not stimulating sleep. A good example is when you are playing with them or they have something that is making them unable to calm down.

Avoid too many errands, noise, toys, and people talking will make your baby overexcited and hence unable to sleep. The solution to this is to create a calm environment for your kids to fall asleep.

3. Physical Discomfort

This is a very common issue that causes the baby to not sleep. Your baby may not be wearing comfy clothes or the beddings maybe rough for them. This makes it extremely difficult for them to fall asleep.

It is advisable to make sure that you find comfy beddings and environment for your kids to fall asleep quickly.

4. The Baby is Too Hot or Cold

When the baby is too hot, they cannot sleep right. Make sure that you set a balanced temperature in their room for them to feel comfortable. If they are too hot, try to wear them light clothing and also if it is cold put them on heavy and warm clothes.

Q2. Where Should My Baby Sleep and At What Temperature?

As we have seen above, temperature greatly affects the sleeping pattern of a kid. Most parents are unaware of what temperature is ideal for their kids and for them to get better sleep.

Some people prefer to sleep together with their kids while others prefer that the kids sleep separately. This is totally good, and there is nothing wrong about it. However, there are some considerations to make;

Somewhere Safe - This is very critical because the safety of your kid should come first. Ensure that your baby is sleeping in a cozy place free from anything that can fall on them. If they are going to sleep on your bed, then you need to make sure that they don't fall on the edges.

According to experts, the safest place for a baby to sleep especially when they are less than 6 months old is in a cot. This should be in the same room as the one you sleep in.

Babies are very poor at regulating their body temperature; therefore, this becomes your responsibility. You should make sure that they are not too cold or too hot. When a baby sleeps in a too hot condition, it increases the risk of SIDS (Sudden Infant Death Syndrome). This is especially common in babies who are one month to 1 year.

Experts recommend that an ideal temperature for the baby should be between 20 to 22.2 .

Q3. What Age Should the Baby Sleep Alone or With Siblings?

This again is another question that a lot of parents ask. Most parents are concerned about when they should let their babies sleep on their own or together with other siblings. This question can be answered simply by a recent study which was published in the Pediatrics. The study revealed that those babies who slept alone at 4 months of age slept longer when they were 9 months of age by 1 hour 40 minutes.

This recent research brings about some contradictions with the already existing recommendations which advise parents to keep their kids in their rooms for the first 12 months.

Our recommendations are to move in stages. This means that you should sleep with your baby close to your bed in a cot. After 6 months, you can move the cot further away in your room (if you have space). This will be the right time to observe the behavior of your kid. Note whether they are comfortable sleeping there and if they fall asleep easily.

Q4. Is My Room Quiet and Dark Enough?

Noise and darkness are a crucial factor to consider when determining whether the room where your baby sleeps is ideal. For one too much noise is definitely not good and your kid might not fall asleep easily and cannot have a sound sleep.

Light and darkness triggers our body and mind and makes them program the sleeping routine. Those individuals who have night shifts at work need to sleep during the day, and the best way to do this is to make sure that the room they want to sleep in is dark.

Q5. Is There an Ideal Sleeping Position for a Baby?

This is another question that parents ask a lot. When your baby is not sleeping the right way, you will begin to ask yourself whether your baby is sleeping in the right way. Actually, there is an ideal sleeping position for kids because some sleeping positions my risk their lives.

The best sleeping practices for kids include:

Make sure that your kids sleep on their back. This is the best position for your baby to fall asleep easily and have a good sleep. This sleeping position was labeled as the best sleeping position for kids by US National Institute of Child Health and Human Development (NICHD).

It is important to pay attention to the beddings and make sure there is not loose bedding which may cover the baby's face. The cot should have a firm mattress rather than a soft mattress.

To make sure that the back-sleeping position is effective, it is recommended that you should keep on turning your baby's head and change the sleeping direction from time to time.

Q6. Should I Let My Baby Cry-It-Out?

CIO is a sleep training technique where you let your baby cry until they fall asleep. This is a highly debated topic which has a lot of critics and proponents among parents. Therefore, there is no simple answer to this question because what works for one parent cannot work for the other.

The goal of this method is to teach your baby to self-soothe before you can intervene and sooth them. It is recommended that you wait for your kid to cry for about 10 minutes and go and sooth them. The following day, it might take less time for them to soothe themselves.

Kid wakes up at night from time to time, and this is completely normal, with this method of cry-it-out, your kid can be able to soothe themselves and get back to sleep after they wake up at night.

Q7. Should I Let My Baby Sleep Through the Night Without Breastfeeding, Bottle-feeding, Or Using A Pacifier?

This is also a critical question that parents ask. Research shows that babies who were born full-term and have no health issues can sleep throughout the night without the need for you to nurse them. There are also some recommendations that you should try to wean the nighttime feeding for your kids at 6 months.

It is recommended that you should discuss the feeding schedule with your doctor before making any changes to a feeding and sleeping schedule of your baby. This is especially important if your baby was born premature or has any other health issues.

Q8. What are Sleep Training Mistakes That Even the Experts Make?

You could be having the right tool for work, but the way you use it determines the success of what you are doing. The same case applies to sleep training. There are so many techniques out there, and parents have used to achieve success in sleep training their kids. Not everything works for everyone, and therefore you need to find what works for you and then go a step further and avoid the following mistakes;

1. Inconsistency

This is one of the biggest mistakes that parents make during sleep training. They fail to be consistent in their sleep training technique. One of the major causes of this problem is tired parents who are unable to be consistent and sometimes even fall asleep.

It is also important to set a good schedule before you begin sleep training. If you are a working parent, you should be able to determine how you will conduct this plan beforehand. Evaluate whether it will be viable or you will end up frustrating your kid or worsen the situation.

2. Extinction Burst

This used to mean that the undesired behavior worsens before it starts to improve when you are getting rid of it. This is a common issue with the sleep training technique such as Cry-it-out".

A good example is when you let your kid cry out for the first night, and it ends up being successful but the second day it gets worse, and they cry too much. Finally, you give up and decide that this cannot work for your kid.

The truth is if you persist, your baby could be done with crying within 3 - 7 days which is usually the average time for "cry it out" technique to work.

3. Starting at the Wrong Time

The best time to start sleeping training is at 6 months. Most parents are desperate about making their babies soothe themselves, and therefore they start too early. This will not do any good but will highly reduce the chances of success in sleep training.

4. Not Paying Attention to Medical Causes of Sleep Difficulties

This is also another serious mistake that people make when sleep training their kids. When your baby has medical issues such as anxiety, pain, asthma, obstructive sleep apnea, and others, they may not respond to any behavioral changes. Therefore, all your effort to get them to sleep better will be futile. It is recommended that you first discuss with the pediatrician about your baby sleeping problem.

5. Destructive Bedroom

This is a common challenge for many parents especially those living in an apartment where there are noises from the streets or neighbors complaining about a child crying. If your kid is sleeping together with their sibling, it can become difficult for the sleep training to be successful. It is, therefore, recommended that you make sure that you have the right room for your kids for the sleep training to succeed.

Now that we have cleared the basics of sleep training and answered the most burning question s about the same, in the next section, I am going to teach you 5 steps to achieve success in sleep training in 5 days.

CHAPTER 2

SECRET FOR LONGER AND BETTER SLEEP FOR YOUR KID AND WHY IT IS IMPORTANT?

Some people may ask, "How long every baby should sleep?"

According to the American Academy of Sleep Medicine, there are ideal hours of sleep that kids should have depending on their age.

For infants who are between 3 - 11 months, they require at least 14 - 15 hours of sleep every day. Toddlers require about 12 - 14 hours of sleep while preschoolers need 11 to 13 hours of sleep every day. All this is inclusive of naps

For you to achieve this for your kids there are a series of practices that you should pay attention to and be consistent in. These include:

1. Make Sure You Establish Healthy Sleep Habits Early

Don't wait for too long to establish a sleeping plan for your kids because the longer you wait, the harder it will be for them to adapt easily.

It is recommended that you establish the plan at the age of 4 months old. Establish an effective to day-night sleeping cycle because this is what will make them have a better and longer sleep.

2. Sleep Hygiene is A Must

Sleep hygiene includes the proper bedtime routine, clean and safe sleeping place, clean beddings, a room free of noise and distractions, ideal room temperature and dim light. With this in place, it will become easier for your kid to fall asleep and remain asleep for long.

3. Set a Sleeping Routine

A routine is very important for its programs or mind and body to automatically move to sleep mode easily. In order to establish a sleeping routine for your kid, you need to ensure that you start by introducing activities or practices that signal to your baby that it is time to sleep. The best way is to have something relaxing before they go to sleep and avoiding distractions and simulations minutes before bedtime. With this, it will become easier for your kids to fall asleep naturally even without your help.

4. Nurse Your Baby Before Bedtime

As they say, A Happy Time = Happy Sleep. When your baby is full, they will tend to sleep better for longer. Make sure that you breastfeed your child minutes to bedtime and let them sleep. For older babies, it is important for you to pay attention to what to give them. Because some food my compromise they sleep.

Be Consistent

All the above secrets to a better sleep require you as a parent to be consistent for you to achieve success. If for example, you are setting a sleep routine for your kid, you need to be consistent failure to do so will lead to a distracted sleeping routine which is not good for your child. Be sure to have a schedule for your kid which you follow strictly, and this will not only make them sleep easily but will help them even when they age.

Reasons Why Longer and Better Sleep Is Important for Your Baby

Sleep is very important for babies especially during their young age. The following is the importance of better baby sleep.

1. Sleep Promotes Growth

Research reveals that growth hormones are secreted during sleep time. This, therefore, increases the need for you to ensure that y our baby is getting enough sleep for them to grow. It is recommended that babies should spend at least 50% of their time sleeping.

2. Sleep Is Good for The Heart

Sleep protects kids from vascular damage. Children with sleep disorders have been found to have excess brain arousal during sleep, and this can be bad for the heart. The blood cortisol and glucose are elevated at night, and this has been linked to an increased level of obesity, diabetes and heart disease.

3. Sleep Increases Attention Span

It has been found out that kids who have less sleep during young age had a tendency of having hyperactivity and impulsive issues when they arc 6 years. Kids who are tired and sleepless get distracted casily and are not attentive. To increase the attention span of your kid, it is important to ensure they are getting enough sleep every night.

4. Sleep Increases Learning Ability

Research from Columbia University Medical Center revealed a baby brain works more when they are asleep. Sleep doesn't not only aid learning in small kids only, but it also helps kids in other ages as well. It is therefore important to make sure that the kids are getting enough sleep in order to promote good learning.

5 Steps to Achieve Deeper Baby Sleep in 5 Days

Did you know that it is completely possible to achieve success in sleep training within 5 days? Your child needs that sleep the same way you need it, it is, therefore, a win-win scenario. Helping your baby sleep better and longer is a process and requires you to take a series of actions in order to succeed. The following are the 5 steps to take to achieve a better sleep for your baby.

Step 1 – Set the stage

Having a consistent environment will facilitate a better sleep for your baby. You should be the one to set that stage before you attempt anything else. According to experts, babies get their best naps and night sleeps in their baby crib. So this means that you've got to start from here.

Make sure that the crib is comfy and clean. The room where you want your baby to sleep should be soundproof. Make sure also that there is no noise so that your baby will sleep better. Consider getting white noise for your baby so that this can diminish other noises that may be present.

Step2 – Start by Planning the Morning First

Remember that your baby needs at least 15 hours of sleep every day. This means that nighttime sleep will not be enough. You have to make sure that you facilitate daytime naps.

The first nap that is very important is the morning nap. This may not necessarily be a long one so don't to worry too much about that because it is just a single sleep cycle.

Afternoon naps are also very important because it helps your kid to be relaxed after they are tired. Day naps should be regulated and you should set up a specific time to facilitate that. This way your kid will fall into the routine of sleeping at that time every day which will help him get better and sound sleep.

Step 3 – Discourage Catnap

Catnapping is common in babies but you should discourage this by making sure that both the morning and afternoon naps are prolonged. This is important and it will help your kid to sleep better and longer during that time.

To ensure that this is effective, do not take them away from their crib. Wait for some minutes and see whether they fall back to sleep again. Leaving them in this sleeping environment will help their brain understand that that time of the day is for sleeping.

Step 4 – Timing is Crucial

Babies of about 4 – 6 months old require 3 naps in a day. One in the morning, afternoon and later before dark. This last nap time usually goes away after some time. It is recommended that the bedtime for babies be around 5 to 7 pm and they should wake up at 6 -7 am. After they wake up, the first nap should start at around 8 – 9 am in the morning. Having this timing is important because once they fall into the system; it will be easier for you to plan your day well.

Step 5 – Give Them Time

Now that you have played your role in ensuring that your kids get enough sleep you should give them time to adapt to this new way of life. It's like learning a new skill, and therefore you need to let it sink. Don't give up or abandon the plan if you see no change after a few days.

Be consistent and don't give up and soon all will work out. Kids respond differently to these changes, and therefore you should know that it might take some time. Never compare your baby with that of your neighbor.

After these steps, you can now go ahead and implement the following in five days. With the following daily action plan, you will achieve success in giving your kid a better sleep in 5 days.

Day-to-Day Actions Plan to Follow for 5 Days

Day 1 - Start a Routine

Day 1: Setting a routine should be the first step to achieving success in better baby sleep in 5 days. This routine should be based on the sleep training method that works for you. As we saw earlier, babies are born confused between days and nights. That is the reason why you will find that they sleep for long in the afternoon and wake up at night to play.

The next thing you need to do is to place your baby cot near a window where there is enough natural light. This will help the baby to have an organized cardiac rhythm.

In the evening of day one, make sure you set a sleeping routine. This starts by creating quiet rituals. You can do this by making your kid have to wear pajamas, lower the volume of your TV, dim the lights and put the child in their crib. This triggers their sensory system to slow down which will facilitate comfortable sleeping.

Day 2 - Practice, Practice

Day 2 should be all about repeating what you did yesterday. Practice makes perfect, and therefore you have to keep on practicing for this to work. If you realize that your kid needs feeding during the night time, you should make sure that you feed them while still aligning to the routine you created.

Be flexible in finding the right thing that soothes your baby to sleep in the evening. You can try out a bath which can either turn out to be calming or invigorating; this varies between kids. Once you establish what works for your kid, you stick to that.

Day 3 - Hitting and Overcoming the First Roadblock

The ultimate goal here is to make sure that your kid can fall asleep alone and to achieve this, you need to do something exciting yet tough.

The last two days, you have been putting your kid in that cot while asleep. In day 3 you should put them in their crib while awake.

This might trigger a cry, but the truth is that this will be tough for you and not your kid. The crying will release some tension in them, and they will eventually fall asleep. This is where it gets tough for most parents because they find it very agonizing to watch their kids cry.

The best thing to do in this situation is to let go the feeling that you will be causing psychological harm to your kid. If you are consistent in this, you will win the battle very soon. You should, however, keep on checking on your baby periodically. You can start with 5 minutes for the first time.

Ensure that you don't turn on the lights, or remove him from the cot or give him a pacifier. If you give them any of this, they will cry the following day, and that is what we want to avoid.

Day 4 - Press On - Baby Settles In

Day 3 will be a hard one, and now we are on day 4, and the good news is that you can expect some improvements. You will repeat the same exact thing you did yesterday. Your baby will now realize that crying bears no results and they will cry less or not cry at all.

In case they cry, you can prolong your response time to about 10 minutes or longer. This is where you have to tough it out and don't give in. If you give up, you will create an opportunity for your kid to cry even more and this will worsen the situation.

Research shows that most babies will get into the system in 3 - 5 days and therefore if you followed all steps above in the right way, day 4 and 5 should be the day you win this battle. However, make sure that you do not change the routine and keep it as it is.

Nigh feeding will be the only challenge but you depending on the age of your kid, you can cut them out or keep them as quiet and as brief as possible. Over-feeding them means that they will mess their diapers and this will keep them awake.

Day 5 - The Baby Sleeps, and You Sleep Soundly Too

This is where it gets interesting. You have created a sleeping routine for your kid in 5 days, and at the same time, you have managed to regain your sleep. Good sleep habit is very critical in for the good health of your kid. It is therefore important to try out ways in which you can achieve better and longer sleep for your kid as soon as possible.

This technique has been tried by many parents and is proven to work. In the next section, we are going to look at the success stories of parents who have used this technique and have succeeded.

Success Stories of Parents Who Used Our Technique and Achieved Sleep Training for Their Kids

Having tried to find a method of sleep training that will work for you without any success is one of the most stressing things you can ever have. However, the technique shared above proved to work for many parents who live to testify and encourage others to try out the technique.

So many people give you just the theory, but they never go a step further to provide you with the exact way you can implement that information. In this book, we have made sure that we provide the exact step by step to make it easy for you to achieve success in sleep training. The following are the stories from those who have succeeded.

Niemeyer

"I was first reluctant to try out the 5 steps 5 days sleep training technique because it seemed to be too far from solving my problem. However, I needed to stop my kid from crying at night, and therefore I decided to use this technique. I made a mistake the first time, but I tried because I was not consistent. I tried the first time and it never worked and my child cried even more.

I again decided to try again and this time around I was serious about it. I also had the support of my wife after I enlightened him about my sleep training plan. The first day was messy, but finally, our daughter slept after 30 minutes of crying. The second day she never cried at all which was like a miracle to us. The rest is history, and it's been 7 months now, and it has been a routine for her.

One thing I would like to advise parents is to be consistent and realize that you should not stop. This is more of a process, and you should not stop after seeing some success. You should be very consistent until it becomes very easy for your kid to fall asleep.

I am looking forward to seeing my daughter go to sleep be herself without forcing her even when she gets old."

Aliana K.

I had searched all over the web, and I never found a lasting solution to sleep problems with my son. I came across the 5 steps in 5 days sleep training technique, and since I was so desperate to get my son to sleep, I followed every bit of instructions.

I was surprised at how effective the technique was. Never ever look for something super serious about sleep training. It's all about the basics and best sleep habits that we are told about every now and then.

Just be a good parent, make sure that your child sleep at a safe and comfy place and the rest is magic."

As Aliana K says, never look for something extraordinary it's the basics that work, and that's exactly what we teach you in this book.

CHAPTER 3

BABY SLEEP TRAINING BONUS EXPERT TIPS

We are not going to leave you at that, but we will give you some expert bonus tips to help you as you embark to this journey of baby sleep training program.

This is important for it will complement your efforts and makes it easier for you and your child to achieve sleep success within the best time possible. These expert tips are also helpful for those who will find it difficult or encounter challenges in the sleep training program.

These tips will not only help your kid to get better sleep but will also keep them comfortable and feeling loved. This section will also teach you the safety issues that you are a parent should know about your kid and the best sleep habits you should adapt to every time.

Tip #1. Useful Baby Gadgets and Massage Techniques

There are so many baby gadgets in the market today. These gadgets are great in simplifying the work of making our kids sleep and keeping them asleep. We will slit this to a different category so that you will know what gadget is right and at what time.

Gadgets for Establishing a Sleeping Routine

As we saw earlier, then the first step to achieving success in sleep training is to establish a routine for your kid. With a routine, it will become very easy for you and your child to fall asleep easily every day. Some of the useful gadgets for setting a sleeping routine for your kid include:

1. Musical Soother

These are singing and dancing sleep gadgets that are effective in creating a bedtime routine for your kids. The gadget cine fitted with soothing sounds which are cool and calming for kids. These can be in the form of melodies and nature sounds.

2. Night Light Projector

This is also another routine nighttime gadget. The gadget reflects colorful stars, lights, and clouds that help your little one to nod off easily.

3. Baby Shuster's

This is an awesome gadget; it works by producing a shushing" sound to soothe your kid. It makes a sound that is similar to you making your kid think that you are still around. It has a timer that allows the shushing sounds to fade away after a set time.

4. Galaxy Clock

This gadget is packed with features that allow good sleeping routine for your kid. It projects stars and produces white noise as well as nature noise creating a sleeping environment for your kid.

The gadget is best in setting a daily sleeping routine for your kid. Using any of these or a combination of some will help you to set the routine for your baby easily and without struggling too much. This is also appropriate for those parents who have a busy schedule.

Gadgets for Keeping Your Baby Sleeping

It can be a huge investment and almost impossible to keep your baby room sound proof. What makes your baby sleep sound is a quiet and conducive environment for your kid. If you have checked that, you can go a step further (but not necessary) and complement by adding soothing sounds and white noise.

All the soothing gadgets that we have seen above can be used to keep your baby asleep.

A baby monitor is an effective tool that can help you avoid going to your child's room too often which can wake them up. There are lots of types of baby monitors in the market today. Select what is appropriate for you. You can go for a more advanced baby monitor which has features such as a thermometer to keep track of room temperature.

Gadgets for Temperature Monitoring

Temperature affects baby's sleep. A too hot or too cold environment is not conducive for your baby to sleep in. It is therefore important to make sure that you keep the room temperature well checked. There are tools for that such as:

Wearable Blankets - This is sleeveless bodysuit designed to keep your baby warm. It has a zipper making it easy to wear comfortably. It is safe to use and doesn't risk your child health or SIDS.

Thermostats - The same way you heat the other rooms of your home, you can hear your child room and ensure that the temperature is the right ones (22.2 degrees Celsius). Using a thermostat and a baby monitor with a thermometer will be a sure way to ensure that your baby sleeps in a well-heated environment.

With the above gadget, you can achieve success in sleep training, and soon you might not need the gadget when the child gets into the sleeping program.

Baby Massage Techniques

There are many benefits of massaging your baby. Each gentle stroke you give your baby makes them feel loved, nurtured and it creates a bond between both of you. Massage in babies helps them to feel more relaxed which aids in improving their sleep.

Benefits of Baby Massage

Baby massage helps in stimulating both digestive and circulatory systems. This, according to International Association of Infant Massage (IAIM), can help deal with conditions such as cramps, constipation, colic, and gas.

Massage relieves growing pains, teething discomfort and muscular tension in babies. All these benefits contribute to a better life of your kid.

When to Start

Most parents wonder when to start to massage their kids but experts suggest that you should introduce touch as soon, they are born. It is advisable to ensure your kid is relaxed and calm before you start massaging them. One sign, when they stiffen their arms or move their head away from you, then they are not ready for massaging.

There is no limit on how often you should massage your baby. Some parents massage their kids in the morning while others do that in the evening before bedtime which promotes easy sleeping.

Techniques for Massaging Your Kid

The following tips will help you have an effective massage for your kid.

Make the Atmosphere Cozy

The massage atmosphere needs to be calm and quiet. Ensure that your baby is in a comfortable place such as on a couch, changing table or your bed. A comfortable environment makes the massage to be effective.

Start Slow

Lay your baby on their back and start by slowly rubbing their body parts gently. It is recommended that you start with their head and proceed down to the feet. Make sure you spend some time on each body parts as long as they are enjoying it. It is important to try placing your baby on their tummy and massage their back. Make sure this is very brief.

Repeat Again

If you see that your baby is enjoying the massage, you can start again from their forehead all the way down.

Talk To Your Baby

Communication during a massage is very important because it creates a bond and further relaxation of your baby. You can even mention their name during the massage, and this will make them feel loved. If your goal is to make them fall asleep, you can sing to them some songs or some nursery rhyme.

Use Some Oil

To use or not to use the oil is optional but it is important because it helps in the reduction of body friction during the massage. Make sure that the oil is not smelly. Also, ensure that you know what is good for your baby's skin especially if they have sensitive skin or allergies.

Baby massage is a great ingredient to their relaxation and will ultimately lead to their sound sleep. Get creative in this and include it to their bedtime routine to facilitate better sleep.

Tip #2. Easy yet Effective Sleep Habits Parents Should Implement Right Away

Effective sleeping habits will increase the chances of success in sleep training. These are easy to follow habits that you can make them like a routine to achieve maximum success.

Create nighttime and a regular sleeping routine for your kids. - From today onwards make sure that you set a routine for your kid and stick to it. Aim at putting your baby to sleep at the exact same time every day. Make sure also that you start your evening routine such as bath, feeding, stories, etc. at the same time every day.

Limit the daytime naps - This is very important because it will help your child to sleep more at night instead of day time. This, however, should be done to kids who are aged 3 months and above.

Avoid Giving Bottles in Bed - This is for safety purpose and also will help your kids to fall asleep without any external assistance.

Place Your Child on His Back - It is safe to let your baby sleep on their back. This is the safest way to ensure that your child does not fall into the risk of SIDS.

Put Your Baby on Be When They Are Not Asleep - This is very important because it will help the baby to learn to sleep on their own.

Ensure the Baby Is Not Hungry - It is important to feed your baby right before going to sleep. When the baby sleeps when full, they will sleep better and longer.

Tip #3. Potential Sleep Regression Management Guide

Sleep regression is a time during the 4-month age of your baby whereby the sleeping pattern shifts. Your baby wakes up at night and is unable to go back to sleep. This is a completely normal condition, and for the newest parent, it can be stressing.

The good news about sleep regression is that they are temporally and is not a must they occur to your child. However, you need to be prepared and be informed of what happens in this condition.

The science behind sleep regression is the developmental milestone such as brain growth. As your baby grows, he continues to adapt to the new environment and new experiences. These experiences and struggles to learn something new are the ones that disarrange the baby sleep patterns.

Some signs of sleep regression include multiple-night waking, changes in appetite, less napping and fussiness.

How to Manage Sleep Regression

Give them time To Practice new Skills - As we have seen sleep regression is caused by your baby's development. As they learn new skills, keep them awake during the day to practice those skills such as sitting up or rolling over.

Feed them During the Day - Make sure that you fully feed your baby during the day. As they are curious about the new experiences and environment around them, they tend to shift their attention from feeding. Making sure they are full will help avoid cases of them getting hungry at night.

Keep the Room Dark - This will encourage them to sleep. You should also make sure that when they wake up in the morning, you let the light slip to their room so that their bran can have a sleep-wake cycle.

Establish a Routine - As we have seen earlier, it is critical to establish a sleeping routine for your kids early enough. By doing this, it will become easier for them and for you to deal with sleep regression when it occurs.

Pay Attention to Sleep Cues - These signs of sleep are important to note so that you can be swift to take action and help them to drift off to sleep fast by placing them in an environment suitable for sleeping.

Tip #4. Sleep Safety Questions Answered

Child safety is very important because babies are young and very sensitive and delicate. It is the responsibility of every parent to make sure that they provide safety for their kids. Sleep safety is a hot topic among parents and in this section; we are going to answer some of the commonly asked questions about this.

Q1. Where is the Safest Place for a Baby to Sleep?

In the parent's bed if it has enough space, in the crib placed in the parents' room. After about 6 months, you can give them a separate room if it's available

Q2. Is it okay to include other beddings in the baby's crib?

It is recommended that the cot have tightly fitting bedding. This will prevent the beddings from rolling over your baby's head covering his nose which can be dangerous.

Q3. What is the Safest Sleeping Position?

The safest sleeping position for your baby is on his back. This will help reduce the risk of SIDS.

Q4. Is it Safe to Place Hanging Toys?

These are safe if they are installed correctly. However, make sure that they are removed when the baby starts to move or when he can reach them. They should be moved higher out of reach of the baby.

Q5. Which Age Should You Stop Back Position for Sleep?

The preferred age to stop back sleeping position for your kid is 1 year.

Q6. Should Soft Sleeping Surface Be Avoided?

It is important to keep away everything that can increase the chances of suffocation.

Q7. Is it safe to use soother or pacifiers?

Research shows that soothers and pacifiers never interfere with breastfeeding. They can also help in getting your baby to fall asleep easily.

Q8. Is room Sharing Safe?

Room sharing is safe if the baby is sleeping separately in their own surface like crib or bassinet. It is recommended that you should share the room with your kid for at least 6 months.

Q9. Is it safe to put more than one Kid in the same crib?

To avoid the risk of SIDS, it is important to get each kid his or her own crib. This will prevent them from getting suffocated or any other sleep-related injury.

Q10. Is it Safe to Feed a Baby lying on the bed?

This is risky especially if you fall asleep and this can be dangerous to your kid. If you feel sleepy, it is important to put the baby back to their crib.

Chapter 4

Summary of the Key Action Plans for Better Baby Sleep

Thank you for making it this far, I hope you have learned a lot of helpful information about sleep training for your kid. In this section, I am going to give you a recap of what we have learned in the previous sections. Use this book as a reference in case you get stuck somewhere. The key action plans to take include:

1. **Realize the Benefits of Sleep for your kids and Give Them What They Deserve**

The first thing you need to do is to understand that sleep is very crucial to the health of your kids. Once you realize that, you will be in a position to give than what they deserve. There are so many conditions that are associated with lack of sleep including poor development and lack of concentration.

Just as much as you love to sleep, you should also make sure that you give your kids an ideal environment for them to fall asleep easily. From today onwards you should set aside a better sleeping place for your kid. The room should be conducive, and the bed should be comfy. Also, make sure that you pay attention to other factors that may limit the sound sleep of your kid such as noise and temperature.

2. Use the 5 Steps in 5 Days Plan to Achieve Better and Longer Sleep for your Kid

Go back to Chapter 2 and familiarize yourself with the 5 steps to achieve better sleep for your kid. This plan is very critical in making sure that you give your kid the sleep they deserve as soon as possible.

The goal is to make sure that the kids can sleep by themselves and this will give you the peace of mind because you too will be able to sleep. When the kids are about 4-6 months, this is the best time to establish a sleeping plan for them. This will not only help them when young but will also help them as they get older without forgetting the so many benefits that come with sound sleep.

3. Avoid the Sleep Training mistakes

Most parents are despaired in creating a sweeping plan for their kids and in this process, they end up messing everything. Look at Chapter 1 and learn about these mistakes and avoid repeating them.

One of these mistakes can have a serious consequence to your kids. It is therefore important to stick to a plan and take things one at a time. Remember consistency and dedication is what will bring about success to any sleep training efforts.

Most parents give up, and they end up in a worse situation than they were in. You should, therefore, make sure that you are ready and dedicated to learning about sleep training for your kid and implementing it.

4. Safety is the key

Always remember that the safety of your kid is in your own hands. You should do everything within your means to ensure that you maintain that. There are so many security questions that most parents ask. You can refer to them again in Chapter 3 to be on the safe side.

If you are unsure of anything, it is important to consult with your pediatrician so that everything will be smooth and you will not risk the health and the life of your kid.

5. No More Wrestling with Your Baby

As a parent, it is your responsibility to adapt to best sleeping habits that will be for the wellbeing of your baby. These sleeping habits are well highlighted in Chapter 3. These form the basis of safe and effective sleep training.

You are in the position to give your child the sleep they deserve. It doesn't have to be as hard as it sounds, it is doing all that you need to do is to go back to this book and use the actionable steps given.

There is no need to wrestle with your kid. You have the solution, and it is your responsibility to make this work. The good news is that you have the information and the exact way to get this done; make it happen today.

Conclusion

Knowing your goals and what you want to achieve and being dedicated to achieving it is what will make you successful in achieving success in sleep training.

There are so many people out there who are struggling to find a solution for their baby sleep. This is what motivated me to craft his guide book to help them. If you are reading this, you are one of them, and I hope it is going to help you. You don't have to use high-end techniques all you need our 5 steps in 5 days sleep training technique.

All the information, tips, guides, recommendation in this book is verified and tested by many. It is, therefore, your turn to implement the information in this book to achieve success in sleep training for your baby.

Take action today, be consistent and within no time you will be happy with the results.

-- *Patrick Bradley*

www.ingramcontent.com/pod-product-compliance
Lightning Source LLC
Chambersburg PA
CBHW051405280526
45784CB00007B/3101